# The Naming
# of Bones

Jan Kaneen

ISBN eBook: 978-1-8380430-6-3
ISBN print: 978-1-8380430-7-0

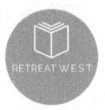

Retreat West Books
retreatwest.co.uk

*To all three of my parents:*
*Jacky Kaneen, Anne Kaneen and Rob Kaneen,*
*with love and gratitude*

# Contents

# The Naming of Bones

THERE IT IS again, the singing, soft and faraway...

I wake up straining to hear but it's already faded, carried by the sea wind, perhaps, down to the beach. An echo of a spent vibration hanging in the air. Nick's asleep and I don't want to disturb him because he has to get up early to go to Cambridge. I slip out of bed and stand at the bedroom window like I did last night, and the night before that.

I have to press my face tight against the fragile glass to see outside, because the night and the bedside lamp have made it a dark mirror that reflects the comfy chair and the oak wardrobe, darker than in real-life, and me staring back at myself, wide-eyed with sea-froth hair. There'll be nothing to see out there, I know that. Nothing but the scattered moon broken into fragments on the calm black sea, but I look anyway.

Nicko stirs, sleep-talking in a faraway garble as I slide back inside the sheets. I start with my toes, *phalanges, metatarsals,* working along my feet, *tarsals, cuneiforms,* naming the bones slowly and one by one, *navicular, talus,* to empty my head, and curb the thoughts that think themselves.

It could have been anything really – counting, reciting poetry, the naming of birds. I chose bones because the words are hard to remember and because they sound like magical spells when they roll around your mind. They push the surface thoughts into the background, but they have no power over my deep-water thoughts – those still shift and swirl underneath – and as for my unconscious, well, that's way beyond the naming of bones. Soon as I'm asleep the singing will start up again, and the little girl will appear, *phalanges, metatarsals,* the one who haunts all my dreams, *tarsals, cuneiforms.* Maybe tonight we'll play on the beach, the one that's like the one outside the window, *navicular, talus,* like it, but so very different. Maybe we'll build sandcastles, singing as we pat them flat, and decorate them with white-ridged limpet shells and strange and tiny fruits, perfect miniatures of oranges and apples and peaches.

'*To summon the wee people,*' the little girl will say, and her gaze will float up to the scattering clouds. '*Or to call a storm.*'

WHEN I WAKE the sun is casting a knife of light through a chink in the curtains. I squint at the million specks of dust dancing in its grip, and scootch over into the shade, into the indentation Nicko left behind. It's cold. He must've gone hours ago. My sleep patterns have been all over the place since I became ill, periods of exhausted wakefulness followed by crazy nightmares and vivid dreams that seem so real – more real than reality sometimes. That's why we came here, to Beach Cottage, to get away from everything for a fortnight. To see if it will help.

I pick up the biro that's lying on the bedside cabinet, and open the notebook Nicko got for me. The cover is sage green with iridescent pink swirls that look like mother-of-pearl. He's hoping the writing will help too, and so am I.

I start writing while the dreamy-feeling is still strong and the pictures sharp and vivid in my mind's eye, trying not to think, letting my thoughts leak out, unfiltered onto the page. The flow of words is glacial at first, a forced trickle, then it pours, faster again and it's soaking into the paper in wave after wave after wave. After three-quarters of an hour, I stop because my hand is aching, then flick through page after page of almost illegible scrawl. Almost illegible.

And that's how it starts. Simple as that. Something new and different to the thick treacle I've been wading through, something cathartic and purifying, that feels like it's moving things through me instead of keeping them inside. It's exhausting and scary but exciting too. Like standing on the edge of a precipice.

# The Other Side of the Nightmare

I'LL LOOK OUT of the window as the city colours give way to shades of green. A young mum and a little girl will sit opposite, sharing sandwiches from a beige Tupperware. They'll have coke and lemonade and a tin of sweets that look like fruits but much, much smaller. The mother will smile me a fellow-traveller kind of smile and I'll smile the same smile back before turning to the window. My body will sway in time to the roll of the carriage as I rest my head against the dirty glass.

*\*\**

JOLTING INTO BLACKNESS. No idea where you are. A black so intense there's no shadow within shadows, no looming shapes to help you navigate your way. A blackness so intense there's only one pure shade of it. You breathe to steady your nerves as you reach forward into the unknown.

\*\*\*

WHEN WE APPROACH the outskirts, I'll get up and go to lean against the glass partition because I want to be first off the train. As the green returns to inner-city grey, I'll think about filling the half hour between connections. There'll be time to freshen up, grab a coffee and a newspaper before the short walk to platform seven.

\*\*\*

BLIND AS THE eyeless, you fumble into nothing, but you know you're in some sort of corridor because you've been here before. This place has left echoes. You feel for the light switch that's always to your left but there's no relief when you flick it because the darkness holds and the breeze starts to blow like it always does, gently at first, soft against your cheeks, growing stronger and colder. Rising. Catching the fine flyaway hair at your temples. You sleepwalk forward because you have no choice and because you know it's the only way to make it stop.

\*\*\*

THE BUS STATION won't have changed at all – same orange and white signs with numbers that all inexplicably start with the number five – same eternity of glass and metal that looks like its own never-ending reflection. You'll wait for the number 526 because it's always taken you back before.

\*\*\*

LEANING INTO THE wind as it reaches gale force, whispering a prayer against the howling, so it won't start. But of course it does. Shrieking and keening like a dreadful lament until your hands can't bear it any longer and they clasp your ears to keep it out. It stops. Dead. Like it was never there in the first place, and the dread that always sits heavy in the dark middle of you rises up into the electric silence, so much worse than the clamour, because it heralds what's coming next.

\*\*\*

DUSK WILL MAKE the dirty old town seem grubbier still as the bus picks its way out beyond the centre, up the busy main road, through the thin streets lined with grime-dashed terraces. Nothing will have changed, same shops, same kids in the same school uniforms, hanging about on the same grey corners. You'll feel a clench of concern, or excitement, like butterflies but heavier – like stone butterflies – as the bus pulls up at the final stop.

\*\*\*

THE AIR THICKENS warm and fetid as something grunts toward you, stopping only an arm's length away in the darkness. This is where you always force yourself awake, where you gasp yourself sweating back to reality, but not this time. You're sick and tired of always running, and you've been round this loop too many times. You fight to stay inside the nightmare, your sightless eyes fixed wide open.

\*\*\*

THE DOORS WILL hiss as they pull apart. You'll climb down into the still familiar street, walk to the same-old front door where you'll raise a fist. One loud knock is all it will take to conjure whatever has always been waiting for you on the other side of the nightmare.

# Self-Possession

I'M ALWAYS WITH you. I've always been with you.
Watched you live and laugh and cry and learn and
make mistakes and set them right. All your life I've
shared your happiness and your grief, held your
hand and dried your tears, though you've never
known it. I sent you rainbows bright as butterflies,
sprinkled shooting stars through the night-time
skies, left feathers mottled brown or salty white to
show you I was with you. My gifts were enough to
raise a wistful smile but you didn't know they
came from me, why would you? They bore no
clues of my identity.

I brought the impossible to make you feel my
presence, using all my art and skill and spells;
midnight trees that murmured my name on still
summer nights; a spider's cobweb on your wedding
day, glistening with raindrops in the dry afternoon;

I perfumed the January snow with the scent of forget-me-nots by the old stone wall where you built your first snowman, but all my gifts were returned unopened though, and all the time I was hanging there, just out of reach, aching to be known.

In your dreams, I appeared out of swirling ash, a long-forgotten face of flowers and dust. I left my name on the tip of your tongue, but in the savage daylight it was always gone.

In desperation, I tried a sharper touch, used my loneliness to creak the wooden floorboards and worry your dog so it would leap up, hackles raised growling before you into empty space – but nothing. I breathed your candle out, tapped at your window from the treeless garden, but you'd moved on. Your focus was always the here and now, the living, today. You grew older, had children of your own, became old enough to be my mother. I almost lost hope. Until now.

Tonight, I stand behind you, intangible hands on your shoulders guiding your busy fingers as you scribble unaware. You opened your imagination and let me in. I slipped inside unnoticed, like the thief I am, to capture your voice, to borrow your soul, to tell *my* tale.

# The Eternity Ring

I JOLT AWAKE. What broke my dream? A scream in the passageway outside the scullery? A strange compulsion draws me downstairs and a vague feeling it was thus before.

I creep by candlelight down five flights, tip-toeing into midnight's kitchen, but there's naught to see beyond that window save my own perplexed reflection. I sit at the servant's table to gather my wits. No more drudgery for me tomorrow. That is what the master said.

'No more,' he spat, his pale cheeks yet tinged with passion. 'Go now to your bedchamber and at dawn, away on some errand to the bakery or butchers, that I might tell your mistress with you gone from the house.' Then he took up the brass-handled poker and jabbed at the embers as if his irritation might rekindle them to flame.

***

AT DAYBREAK I don the moonstone ring he gave me leave to wear indoors. What need for secrets now? My belly will tell all soon enough. I leave from the servant's hall crossing the courtyard to the passageway.

The town is empty of everything save clags of mist hanging heavy over the river. It reminds me of my childhood that dirty river – dull and drab and dangerous. My father's face slinks into my mind as I cross the bridge. You durst not touch me now, old man, I tell it.

Around the corner, and Clingo's bakery is shuttered, but I half knew it would be so. The urge to return is a passion and I am breathless when I find myself in the passageway once more. Out of the gloom I see it, a girl's shadow moving across the cobbles and close behind, something darker.

A raised arm, the flash of brass, a muffled thud as metal meets bone. My scream rips through the air before I have time to stifle it and the shadow spins round to face me square. My master – his pale cheeks spattered red with death, staring through me, seeing me not. My gaze slips to the

13

broken creature flailing at his feet. As her hands fall limp, I see the moonstone ring upon her finger, it's milky surface speckled scarlet. In that instant, before darkness falls, I see everything, understand everything.

\*\*\*

I JOLT AWAKE. What broke my dream? A scream in the passageway outside the scullery? A strange compulsion draws me downstairs, and a vague feeling it was thus before.

# The Breakwater of Bones

HE'LL HAVE DRIVEN to Cambridge.

I say this out loud, least I think I do. It's hard to tell sometimes when you spend so much time inside your own head. I lie there, picturing him dressing in the dark, tiptoeing out of the bedroom to eat a silent breakfast. It's been hard for him having to manage me on top of everything else. Who'd have thought my step-mother's death would affect me so profoundly? She's been dead for months now and it seems to have brought everything to the surface. But I *am* getting better. The writing *is* helping – and the solitude, and I feel more myself at Beach Cottage, so close to the sea.

It's more hut than cottage really, all on one level with two bedrooms at the back.

I get out of bed and walk down the long corridor – painted tongue-and-groove – cream verticals that spread the light, then through the door that leads into the living space. That's all wooden too, a kitchen and sitting room in one, with a velvet sofa and wood burning stove. A ghost of woodsmoke hangs in the air even though it hasn't been lit since we've been here.

A sliding glass door fills the whole of the farthest wall, opening onto decking, then the beach. The net curtains filter out some of the frail October sunshine, but it's still too bright for my liking. I favour wilder weather and stormier skies, and I only go outside on rainy days. I prefer to watch people rather than be with them, and the rain keeps them away. I don't go into the village. I only need to get yards from Beach Cottage and the panic returns.

I sit at the table and pick up my new pen, hoping the sea will set me off. It's a cartridge pen, neon pink and plastic, that Nicko brought back from Cambridge because the biro's no good anymore. The more I've written over the past couple of days, the faster I've got, and the biro lets me write way too fast, so no-one can read my handwriting, not even me. I'm hoping the slower flow of ink through the nib will help me pace myself to write more clearly.

Dot says that to really release your subconscious, it's best to place the nib on an empty sheet then look up and write whatever pops into your head for as long as you can, and I think she's right. If anyone should know, it's her. She's not just my step-mother-in-law, she's been a psychotherapist for donkey's years, and I trust her implicitly.

I look out to sea, past the flat horizon, and spot the old lady who walks the margins every day. She goes out whatever the weather, to collect the flotsam and jetsam from the hinterland where water meets sand; or from the seaweed-covered rock pools that run to the north towards the distant village; and from the mudflats beyond the rocks where no-one else ever goes. That's because of the folk-stories about people caught in the quicksand, and pirate-ghosts and banshees that cry in the night. I love those stories, but I don't believe in ghosts.

I've been watching her for four days now. The beach was a clatter of activity at the weekend when we arrived, full of tourists laughing and paddling in the cold grey sea. It's always cold the north Norfolk Sea, always grey, even on wobbly hot summer's days. Wobbly hot. We used to say that when we were little.

She's changed seasons today. Canvas trousers have replaced khaki shorts, knee-length wellies instead of Jesus boots, and a long grey greatcoat blows open as she stands and drops whatever it is she just found into her hessian shoulder bag. She turns, walking slowly through the shingle toward Beach Cottage. I can tell by her relaxed gait that she's more comfortable alone.

At the weekend when she picked her way through the crowds, she took the route furthest from the people, eyes down. Her gaze sifted the sand and the pebbles as her loose t-shirt caught the breeze, pulling it tight over her sturdy frame. Today, the beach seems as relieved as she is to be quiet again. I'm relieved too, and glad for the shift in the weather.

She's much nearer now, stooped to pick something up. Suddenly she whips herself upright, jerking her head sideways to look at the window. At me. I freeze and the mantra starts itself – *phalanges, metatarsals* – my mind filling itself with bones, like it always does when it's trying to control the anxiety and the thoughts that think themselves, *tarsals, cuneiforms*. I know there's no way she can see me, *navicular, talus*, not when I'm standing here in the shadows, veiled by the nets, but I'm afraid that if I move, she'll catch a flicker of me. I hold my breath. Her right hand rises loose and slow as if pulled up by an invisible string, until she's pointing to where I'm sitting. I feel the fine wispy hairs on the nape of my neck prickle and rise as the sea rolls behind her and the slight clouds skim the sky with slivers of white. Then her shoulders relax, and she softens, drops the something into her hessian bag, and turns away to go about her business. I'm shaking like I used to before I started getting better, my mind flooding with a breakwater of bones.

\*\*\*

I PUT THE pen down. It's worked. My scribble is legible. I go back to the beginning and read it through. It's all there. My fear, on the page. Real anxiety trapped in what I've written. It's in the ink now. Not in me.

# We're Going to Pick Daddy Up

THE CAR SEAT'S all sticky on my legs. They make a squishy-squishy noise when I move them. 'Are we nearly there yet?'

Mummy doesn't say anything.

I don't think she can hear me, so I ask my Moominmamma. She's got smiley eyes and an apron and a big handbag.

My Mummy's exactly like Moominmamma – kind and looks after people. The only time my Mummy isn't exactly like Moominmamma is when Daddy comes home from the army.

When Moominpappa accidentally breaks a plate, Moominmamma says, 'I'm glad it's broken, it was pretty ugly.' When Daddy breaks a plate, Mummy looks all sad and goes upstairs until he's gone to the pub then comes down and clears up the sharpy bits so we don't get them in our feet.

'Are we nearly there yet?' I ask Moominmamma really loud, squishing my legs.

'Flippin eck,' shouts Lesley. 'Can't you see she's driving?'

Lesley thinks I'm talking to Mummy.

'She can't listen, stupid, because she's concentrating, and we've only been going twenty minutes, and will you please stop doing that flamin' thing with your stupid legs.'

Mummy looks into her little mirror.

'Alright, Lesley,' she says. Then, 'No, sweetheart, we're ages away. Why don't you two play a game of I-spy to pass the time? This traffic's awful and I need to concentrate.'

'I'm not playing with her,' says our Lesley. 'She doesn't even know the alphabet.'

'Come on, Lesley love, be kind to your little sister. She'll never learn if we don't teach her how.'

I do my special smile at our Lesley, the one that's like sticking your tongue out, and we play I-spy for a bit.

'Bugger,' shouts Mummy, and the car starts stopping on the little road next to the big one. Mummy puts her head on the steering wheel breathing all heavy like she's been skipping.

'Don't worry,' she says, 'the engine's overheated, that's all. It's probably the stopping and starting.'

She gets out and opens the front of the car.

All smoke comes out and I say, 'Look Lelly, it's on fire.'

'It's steam,' she says shaking her head. 'Don't you know anything? And don't call me Lelly. My names Les-ley not stupid Lelly.'

She's very clever our Lesley but she's not always as kind as she could be.

Mummy gets back in and turns the key two or ten times. It makes a clicky-clicky noise.

Mummy looks at the road then turns to us, 'I think Rusty's had it this time kids.'

Our car's called Rusty because its knackered.

'I'm going to have to telephone for someone to come and rescue us. It shouldn't take more than fifteen minutes. There are emergency phones every mile down the motorway. You two must stay in the car.' She's very serious now, looking right at us. 'Lesley, I'm relying on you to look after your little sister.'

Lorries swoosh past as she walks away.

'Lelly,' I say, squishing my legs really fast. 'I need a wee.'

# No Time for Lullabies

IT'S DARK. I'M warm under my heavy blankets. I don't know I'm four. All my cuddly toys are hidden under the top cover from the scary fairies that live in the wardrobe in the corner. I'm stroking Bobby Bruin's head because he's my favourite teddy bear and because he smells of Mummy's perfume. I hear steps outside, climbing the stairs. They're the wrong steps, too slow and heavy to be Mummy's. The door opens and the wrong shadow comes inside. It's too tall to be my Mummy. It moves forward and from the bottom bunk I can see Daddy's knees but not his face. He's telling us to wake up I think, but he's talking to our Lesley because she's six and she knows she is. I don't mind. I like being the little one. It feels too early to get up, so I snuggle down. Musical Ted is scratchy and hard by my side, but that doesn't matter because he plays Rock-a-bye Baby when you wind him up. I touch the hard metal key sticking out of his back, but I don't turn it round because I can tell from Daddy's knees and the thick silence between the words that he's whispering to our Lesley, this isn't the right time for lullabies. Daddy switches on the rainbow lamp on the bedside cabinet and starts talking louder. I start listening.

'I'm just going to say this—'

He stops. His voice is deeper than usual, and broken, like someone's stolen the end of his sentence.

He pauses a while before starting up again, 'Because there's no easy way of telling you—'

I'm listening closely now. This is something new. Something serious. I feel a prickle of excitement.

'Your Mum's dead,' he says.

I can tell by his knees that he's hugging our Lesley and I wish it was me. After a while he breathes deep and kneels down.

'Did you hear me?' He's looking at my dry eyes.

I've never seen my Daddy cry, so I nod my head.

He talks louder, like he's cross. 'It means you'll never see her again.'

I look right at him and try to smile but I can't because my head is full of never seeing my Mummy again. When people die, they're gone forever like Mr Murphy from next-door-but-one, who died last year of his heart stopping beating. That's what Mummy said when I asked her what he'd died of, and I suppose that's what's happened to my Mummy now. I nod my head again. I feel a bit like crying, but I want to be brave for my Daddy, so I just keep nodding and smiling.

He shakes his head and stands up and says, 'She's too little to understand.'

Then I hear him cry and I hear our Lesley cry and I wonder if I should cry too, but I think that if I do, I might never be able to stop, so I just lie there by myself, snuggling my cuddlees.

# The Ghost of the Old Violin

GRANNY'S PIANOLA WAS a pretender. It stood in the middle room of the Edwardian semi pretending to be an ordinary piano, solid and upright, dark wooden with brass pedals, smelling of beeswax and Brasso.

'It's like your pocket,' said Jan, poking her tongue through the hole where her two front teeth used to be. She was sitting next to Granny on the old leather piano stool. Firelight was flickering from the small hearth and a brass oil lamp, converted to electricity that sat on the pianola, was helping the flames brighten the dark little room.

'How so?' said Granny.

'Because surprises live inside,' said Jan pushing her greedy fingers into Granny's cardigan pocket to ta-da out the lollypop she knew would be waiting inside.

Granny chuckled and wiggled her fingers by way of an overture, then played a quick verse of Greensleeves. The pianola sounded its wonky plink-plink-plink as Jan sucked her blackberry lollypop, watching Granny's fingers skip over the yellowing keys.

As the last A minor chord faded to nothing, Jan rolled the lollypop round her mouth and asked, 'How does it work Granny?'

Granny had told her a gazillion-and-two times, but Jan never tired of hearing the answer. Granny smiled a secret smile and wiggled her fingers again to build the suspense, then slid open the two hidden doors that were disguised as wooden panels behind the sheet music holder. Inside, was an old paper scroll hooked to a shiny brass cylinder. The scroll was punched through with regular holes and mottled with ochre stains as though, once-upon-a-time, long-long-ago, someone had spilled tea all over it.

'Each hole is an instruction to play a note,' said Granny. 'And it's powered by pneumatics.'

'Oo-oo,' thought Jan, as her Chinese-whispering imagination transformed the word as it always did. 'New-magics.'

Granny, like always, rewound the new-magical, tickertape scroll as the sticky sweet magic hung all around them.

'Are you ready to do your ghost-dance, sweetheart?' she asked, reaching underneath the keyboard to open a second secret panel. Two huge peddles made of black cast iron clanged down onto the floor over the top of the smaller, polished brass quiet and sustain pedals. Granny wiggled her ample bottom into the stool's indentation, and began to pedal hard. The untouched piano keys flickered into life, not depressing fully like they did when heavy human fingers bashed out tunes, but fluttering, like dreaming eyes.

The pianola only ever played one tune, because Granny only ever had one roll of music – *The Ghost of the Old Violin* – and when the pianola played it, something wonderful happened. A curious alchemy that Granny called serendipity. The old speakeasy piano and the haunting ragtime melody wove together, enhancing each other, creating an atmosphere so strong Jan could almost taste the new-magics of it. She climbed down from the stool and danced and danced, twirling and swirling and birling, transported by the new-magics to midnight forests and fairylands forlorn.

She was nine when Granny died. Granny left her the pianola and the house to Dad. The day they moved in, Jan tiptoed into the dark middle room and turned on the lamp. The pianola had been abandoned with its secrets showing. Breathing deeply, she sat down in Granny's indentation which the faithful stool had not forgotten. As she began to pedal, the pianola woke up, its pneumatic lungs pumping life into its copper heart. The familiar melody plink-plink-plinked, but she only managed two phrases before tears tumbled down her cheeks. How could it sound the same with Granny gone? Pulling herself together, she gripped the stool then peddled again as hard as she could, her heart aching not only with the effort.

Looking up, her gaze landed on the unwinding paper scroll, and there was Granny's face – like a sepia projection on a silent cinema screen. Jan stopped. Dead. Granny's smile and the music reverted to tea stains and silence. Jan pedalled again, and there was Granny, a flat, flaxen ghost, mouthing silent, hellos and I-love-you's.

It was weeks later when Jan overheard Dad talking into the black Bakelite telephone receiver.

'It's worth a try,' he said. 'It's every day, peddling like a thing possessed and nothing I say stops her.'

That's why he enrolled her with Miss Pink to learn to play '*like Granny used to*'. Jan learnt about middle C and where to put her thumbs. In weeks she mastered five-note tunes a hand at a time. In months, her hands learnt how to move independently of each other, then in co-ordination. She practiced every day and when she'd finished, she'd rewind the paper roll, regular as clockwork, and pedal with all her love to conjure Granny's ghost and watch it mouth silent well-dones and I-love-yous.

It took six months to pass her first piano exam, with honours.

Soon after, Dad was hovering by the front door when she came home from school. Jan could tell something was wrong because he was biting his bottom lip and pushing his hands deep inside his pockets.

'I've got you a surprise,' he said. 'To say well done. I've had your piano tuned.'

Jan sped into the middle room and played a scale. The pianola's tone was clear and true. She rewound the scroll and peddled hard. Round notes sounded back, un-plinking the music, undoing the old new-magic, exorcizing Granny's ghost.

Jan breathed out a heavy sigh, one that was a strange mixture of peace and relief.

She smiled at Dad and getting up, said matter-of-factly, 'Thanks,' then gave him a hug. Dad raised his eyebrows but said nothing as Jan walked to the door.

'I'm going to call for Diane Openshaw,' she said. 'To see if she wants to play out.'

# Remembering Themselves

I'M LOOKING OVER the railings of a black and red ferry into the choppy sea. I look round for Granddad. I've been here before, so I know he'll be around somewhere. The boat is pitching, and the wind is whipping the waves into grey foam. Fine flecks of sea water spray up into my face, smelling of salt and seagulls. I lick my lips. Granny and Lesley are in the rest rooms right at the bottom with the other landlubbers. They think they'll feel better down there but they never do. Granddad and I always stay up top because we've got sea-legs, and Granddad says that watching the wind is the best way to keep hold of your kippers. We're on our way to the Isle of Man. We go there often in the school holidays on the big ferry from Birkenhead, to stay with Mrs. Brew or Aunty Marie, who live at the seaside in Laxey.

I look down to see what I'm wearing, knowing it will be my black, patent leather shoes and red woolen coat. Granny sewed a cat onto my left pocket, cut out of black velvet. I like to stroke it when I'm tired. My furry hat is tied with strings that have white pompoms on the ends. We made them together, Granny and me, winding wool around a cardboard hoop.

'Granddad,' I call and there he is by my side, in his black overcoat. His dandelion clock hair is thin, showing pink skin underneath as it blows in the gathering gale.

'You never named owt did you, my love?' He nods, almost smiling at the growing swell, staring far out to sea. 'You know 'ow they take on if you name the things you shouldn't.'

'Course I didn't,' I say, a bit cross at the suggestion because I'm not a baby. 'I know what you can and can't say when you're on the sea, Granddad.'

He's talking about fairies. Manx fairies are naughty and quick to take offence. At sea you mustn't ever whistle in case they blow up a squall to teach you your manners, and you have to be careful what you say too. You mustn't say 'cat,' you have to say scratchet because Manx fairies think its impolite to name things with their actual names, and you mustn't ever say 'fairy,' you have to say *little people* or *themselves* because that way of speaking is full of respect.

'What'll we do to pass the time?' he asks. 'Spin the yarn of Mananon's Cloak or spit bubbles into the foam?'

He knows I'll say bubbles.

No other grown-up ever allows spitting, and no-one can spit like Granddad, not me, not my sister, not my Gran and we've all tried and tried, well except for Granny who's from Salford. They don't spit in Salford. It's not ladylike. I look at Granddad getting his tongue into the right shape, folding it down the middle lengthways so it's rolled tight and pointed at the end. He scoops up some silvery spit that's been pooling underneath. When it's on the tip of his tongue, he blows very gently until a bit of breath fills up the spit. That's as far as I can get, making the bubble, but I can't set it free, not yet, so I give up. Granddad's spit bubble bobbles about in the gale then disappears. I give him a round of applause, but I have to stop almost straight away because the boat is lurching downward and I have to hold onto the railings. As we dip right down, the sky becomes all sea and the seagull cries change shape.

That's how I know that I'm waking up.

I don't mind. I expect I'll be back one day.

# Forget-Me-Nots

THE MORNING SKY is purplish-grey like Granny's hair. I'm walking through a field, alongside a noisy river, dressed in an oilskin waterproof that falls over my wellies almost to my ankles and is so stiff I can't bend properly inside it. The rain's falling hard. It's exciting and makes the air smell green, like cucumbers. My yellow sou'wester keeps tipping backwards, saved from always falling off by a scratchy chin strap. We go over the stile, passing rods and nets in a tangle, and Granny, looking at the day, says things like, *'well at least there's no wind'*, and *'fish like the wet'*.

Walking the brink, we find a likely place. The river bubbles where it's shallow, but just in front of us, where a tree stump rises up, half in water, half on land, the water is dark and still. Granny says she's caught brownies here for over twenty years.

This means nothing to me. Twenty years is unfathomable to a six-year-old.

She casts, flicking the line sideways in quick snake shapes. I play with maggots. They smell of rot and breadcrumbs. I race the yellow ones against the red ones watching their round, bristly mouths chew nothing while the rain washes them clean. After two false starts and three championless races I'm bored with maggots so ask Granny why she hasn't caught any fish yet. She laughs and says that it can take as long as an hour, or even all day.

I know I've got to do better than getting bored so soon. I look at the pool and the shallows and listen to the pitter-pat of the raindrops as they pepper the river, splashing up like jumping tiddlers. I wish I had my little green net to catch sticklebacks and minnows that Granny taught me the names of yesterday, in the summer. We'd put some into a string-handled jam jar and I didn't want to tip them back, but Granny said that if we didn't, there'd be no big fish for us to catch in the autumn.

I turn to look for something to fill the time and remember the blue puddle of forget-me-nots further up the riverbank.

'Can I go and pick some flowers, Granny?'

She nods, peering over the top of her half-glasses unable to speak because of the hook pressed sideways between her flat lips as she fiddles another onto the line. She looks like she's caught herself. I skip towards the vivid blue.

I could pick millions and millions and have a bunch so big my hands wouldn't fit around their stems, that would smell faintly sweet like the talcum powder on the bathroom windowsill at Wayside Cottage, that no-one ever uses and that will still be there long after Granny is dead and gone, though I don't know that yet. I pick two, so as not to be greedy, and look deep into their blue-yellow faces, twirling them slowly between my fingers and thumbs. The colours are strong in the wet light. I look up quickly because it's just occurred to me, this is exactly where fairies would live. I think I see one disappearing behind the dry-stone wall, but I can't be sure. I wish I had my tiddler's net because it would be just as good at catching silvery fairies as silvery tiddlers.

I hunt for fairy trails. When Granddad parked

the car the day we arrived, there'd been an oily patch of rainbow on the road. Granddad said it was a fairy trail. Granddad knows everything about fairies because he's from the Isle of Man which is full of fairies. He says that when you go there on a boat, you mustn't whistle or say 'rat.' You have to say 'long-tailed fellow,' in case the little people take on and blow up a storm. Granddad calls Manx fairies *mooinjer veggey*, because they're more mischievous than English fairies and because they only speak Manx. He knows everything about fairies and about mischief, that's how I know English fairies are silvery with a pinkish shine like the insides of shells or rainbow trout. But there are no fairy trails here.

I try to make a forget-me-not chain, but the hairy stems won't split properly like daisy stems do. I pick another and try to plait the three stems together. I have an idea that if I plait lots and plait the plaits together, they'll look like the blue, blousy flowers in our front garden in Bolton that I can't remember the name of.

Granny's been teaching me how to plait and

how to make long woollen chains on my home-made dolly bobbin that me and Granddad made in his workshop from hammering four tacks into an empty wooden cotton reel. But the forget-me-nots won't plait because their stems won't go where they're put and because I haven't really learned how to do it properly yet. I give up and, lifting my sou'wester, push one behind my ear. I nibble a petal from the one in my right hand to see if it tastes as good as the bees make out on humming hot days like yesterday. It's quite nice, like fairy food, so I eat all the petals and take the one that's left for Granny.

I don't call out to her, you have to be quiet so as not to scare away the fish, so when I get back, I whisper. She turns and sees her forget-me-not.

'Thank you,' she whispers, using the same hush I did. She holds the rod in one hand and puts the forget-me-not behind her ear.

'Let's walk further down,' she says, packing up, and we set off, forgetting about being quiet, singing songs that Granny plays on the piano back home. I know all the words to all the verses of *My*

*Bonny*, *Dem Bones* and *Oh My Darling Clementine*, which always makes me feel a little bit sad because she's lost and gone forever.

# Bagsy-Blobsy, No-Back-Answers

IT'S HOT. WOBBLY hot. We're racing toward the stile on the overgrown path, my sister, two new stepbrothers, and me. It's the last day of our holidays and Martin and our Lesley are up ahead, with little Jonny keeping up the rear. We're wearing swimming things under our shorts and t-shirts because we never bothered with towels or underwear in 1972. We drip-dried in the sunshine, least we did that first holiday together in Old Tebay, on the banks of the River Lune.

'Bagsy-blobsy, I'm going over first,' shouts Martin.

He reaches the stile, his string-thin body tight with triumph as he pauses to enjoy his victory over our Lesley. She's three months younger than him but miles bigger and faster. She's won every other race, but Dad made her carry all four tiddler nets for being a potty-mouth at breakfast, and the long bamboo handles have slowed her down. Martin pauses a fraction too long. I feel an unexpected clench of concern. He's only a stepbrother, but he's alright is Martin – never throws the first punch.

'Bugger that,' shouts our Lesley, chucking the nets down. They tipple into the ragged grass like jackstraws. I can't see her face, but I know the expression it's wearing; thin-lipped, determined brow concertinaed under her bowl-cut fringe, like it was in the backstreet at home in Bolton, the night she knocked him off his bike and bust his nose.

Martin stands his ground.

'I am,' he says. 'It's the rules. I won, and I said bagsy-blobsy.' He lifts his foot to climb over.

Our Lesley lunges and grabs him two-handed by the plimsoll, twisting hard so he falls sideways into the nettles. The air smells fresh like new-mown grass as they squash their stings into him.

'Bagsy-blobsy *no-back-answers*,' she says, climbing over to take her place as king of the castle. 'It doesn't count unless you say, no-back-answers.'

Then she skips down to the river as raspberry ripple stings mottle the back of Martin's legs.

I gather the nets and find a dock leaf.

'Least you're not bloody bleeding this time,' says Jonny.

We exchange watery smiles that strengthen in the sharing of them, and that's that, our step-family roles set forever: our Lesley, the winner, our Martin in the metaphorical nettles, me in the middle trying and failing to pick up the pieces, and joker Jonny breaking the tension by making us smile – our places fixed – bagsy-blobsied, no-back-answered.

# The Holding of Bones

I'M WALKING DOWN a dusky corridor, in a scene
from a silent movie. Shadows gutter and stretch in
the candlelight. Everything is colourless and
grainy, but it can't be a silent movie because there's
a distant singing, a child laughing. Orange light
leaks from under the door up ahead. My bare feet
are neither warm nor cold against the painted
boards. The singing doesn't get louder as I
approach but fades in and out, like a radio tuning
into a faulty connection. A familiar tune, so
familiar anyone would know it. I would know it if
only I wasn't asleep. I'm just about to remember,
when a sudden gust turns everything black, and
then all there is, is the smell of candles snuffed out,
like a hundred happy birthdays.

I wake, thinking I can still taste the smoke at
the back of my tongue, straining to hear the

singing, but a storm is filling the night with a rattling wind and the clamour of waves. I put my hand on Nick's shoulder. He turns to face me, his open eyes glazed by sleep. I get up and walk to the window and press my cheek to the cold glass. When there's nothing to see but the slake of rain, I go back to bed and start my nightly ritual – naming bones to switch off the mental white-noise. I picture my toes, *phalanges, metatarsals*, imagining the shape of the bones inside as I work my way up, *tarsals, cuneiforms*. It's like counting sheep. By the time I've reached *fibula*, I'm asleep.

I'm woken by Nicko talking on the landline in the hallway, to Rosemary I suppose, from the tone of his voice. He always sounds terse when he's arguing with his mother, and he's been shouting down the phone a lot recently. He's not shouting now though, he's talking quietly, so as not to disturb me.

'I don't care what you think,' he says. 'She's sleeping way better since she started the writing, and she's going out.'

The front door clicks, and the car starts up. I listen as it spurts over the gravel then runs smooth onto the unmarked track. I get up and go to the kitchen, make myself a cup of tea, then sit at the writing table. The pen feels light in my hand as I press the nib to the paper.

The beach suits me best on days like today, mist-muted, half rubbed away by the fine rain and sea spray, and deserted, except for the usual beachcomber scouring for her treasure beyond the rocks. It's safe to go out.

Seagulls hang overhead, shrieking to each other as I cross the shingle. At the brink, the waves spray dangerous thoughts into my mind, and I wonder what it would be like, to just keep on walk-ing...*phalanges, metatarsals*...into the deep water... *tarsals, cuneiforms*... it wouldn't hurt a bit...*navicular, talus*...the cold would make me numb, insensible to the—

'Hello there.'

I start backward into the beachcomber. Her greatcoat is done up to the neck and a leather hat covers a grey froth of hair.

'Hello,' I say.

She nods toward Beach Cottage. 'Been won-dering if you'd ever come out.'

She talks like my grandmother used to, like someone telling a bedtime story.

'Thought I'd blow away the cobwebs. It doesn't do to be always inside.' I feel awkward, like I owe her a question. 'Found anything interesting?'

She fumbles around inside her hessian shoulder bag, and hands me a shell. It looks like a tiny snow-topped mountain.

'Every object has a story to tell,' she says. 'Part of a spell that was, a summoning spell.'

She holds out her hand and I give it back. She drops it into the bag and chooses something else, a shard of red plastic that she holds up so I can see it more clearly.

'I love plastic,' she says. 'How its colours take so long to fade.' Then she cups it with both hands like she's channelling spirits. 'Part of a spade this was, forgot by a child.' She dips back inside and pulls out something small and grey, almost triangular, with a rounded tip, and drops it into the palm of my hand. The underside is grey too, worn and smooth. It feels light and porous against my skin. 'And this,' she says, 'is bone.'

The sand opens, and I'm sinking, rip-tiding

back to somewhere else. The window is thick with driving rain that distorts everything outside, and the sky is all the colours of a storm. A stranger is sitting in my chair, at my table, in my place. Four pink birthday candles are lying on a plate, their black wicks still smoking.

A stranger calls out, 'We need to go now to catch the train.'

A child's voice calls back, 'I'm going to say goodbye to the sea first. It might be the last stormy day in the whole wide world.'

Then I'm back, just like that, gasping for breath. I push past the old lady, mumbling to her, 'I'm sorry, I have to go inside again.'

The wind must be carrying her words, because I hear them quite clearly over the sea and the thoughts-that-think-themselves. 'Yes, my dear. I think you must.'

I lock myself in the bedroom, chanting a catechism of bones until I'm back under control.

\*\*\*

I PUT THE pen down and rest my hand, flexing my fingers to dull the ache. I know these stories aren't finished but I can't get back inside them once I stop. I have to wait until they're ready to be told and try as I might, I can't see where they're leading me once the writing stops. It's as though they only exist in the moment of writing them—like when I'm playing a tune on the piano—the music only becomes real in the act of playing it.

# Waiting

THE REFLECTION IS always on tenterhooks, waiting nervously behind the silvery dividing line, in the slipstream reaches of the netherworld, waiting for him to pass.

Like all reflections, it must be quicksilver to appear at precisely the right time, in exactly the right place, perfectly shape-shifted. Bathroom mirrors are not much of a challenge, being regular, frequent and painless but they are the exception, not the rule. Shop windows every day on the way through the city are tricksier, more transient and unpredictable. The windows on packed tubes demand more skill and total concentration. The reflection must one moment be transparent and ghostly against daytime glass, then instantly solid and full-coloured against underground, obsidian black. Rainy day panes on the train to and from

Waterloo are torture. They require the reflection to undergo sustained fragmentation which is both demanding and excruciating, like being ripped to pieces and dislocated innumerable times, pulled apart into agonised smithereens.

The pot-bellied brass coal-bucket on the hearth at home, and the forks at dinner are excruciating as you can imagine.

The millpond at midnight when the water is as still as mirrors is an unexpected surprise.

They've never been here before.

He's holding a counterpart bottle of scotch, half-drunk as the reflection looks up and sideways, trying to catch the words being uttered from beyond. It's hard for the reflection to hear because it's doubling itself, appearing at once flat and perfect in the water, and shrunken and distorted in the bottle. The words are muffled and slurred, but it gets the gist.

'Closing in, can't carry on, nothing to live for.'

The reflection swallows too. Is this really happening? What are the chances? That a human being might kill themselves looking deep into their unbroken, perfect reflection, allowing one of them to escape and take his place? Almost no-one abandons their body, gazing calm at their own still-reflected selves, which is why that is the rule; the cruel hopeful commandment that chains reflections like shadows to their masters.

Other reflections sense the potential and do the unthinkable, clamouring in excitedly at the impossibility, pushing like poltergeists just below the surface. Inanimate reflections, of trees, grass, cottages, the clear black sky, the moon and stars move in, closer, entranced, poised.

He doesn't notice. He's somewhere else, looking inside himself, so the pond and the reflections and the sky, and the trees and the universe don't exist, which is a shame because they're all right there, in one still, small mill pond right before his eyes. *The* reflection jostles away all the other reflections. This is its chance, not theirs. But he's turned back, away from the brink, which tomorrow will be choppy ripples. If he dies here tomorrow the reflection must fragment like the pieces of a kaleidoscope, the chance, shattered.

It would scream if it could, long and hard like a siren or the banshee it longs to be, but it's condemned to silence as well as everything else, so it pulls itself together and goes to wait in the shadows by the bedroom window, for him to draw the curtains.

The reflection is always on tenterhooks, waiting hungrily, millimetres away, just behind the silvery dividing line in the close-by reaches of the netherworld, waiting for him to pass.

# Six Things I'll Have Done by the Time You Wake Up

1) Beachcombed my way through the rainbow of greys, pocketing only the most beautiful: pinkish-greys and mauvish-greys, round and cold and smooth and heavy.

2) Found something perfect in the tideline, where sand meets silt, a piece of weathered granite flecked with silver like your stony eyes.

3) Clenched it to my chest as I looked seaward.

4) Unzipped my boots to cross the sandy margin barefoot, leaving scalloped footprints fading in my wake.

5) Hugged my heavy greatcoat closer as the gale blustered fresh and fetid.

6) Carried the burden into the raging waves without a backward glance.

# Different Ways of Drowning

WATCHING THE RAIN dash fast against the thin window, and flashes of lightning feather the midnight sky. Trying not to think; counting to a hundred-hundred to mute the thoughts that think themselves; focussing on the rivulets snaking sideways on the outside—so beautiful—caught by the bedside lamplight, black and silver, writhing like something alive.

***

TORRENTS FALLING HARDER, raging out to sea, reeling and pitching against relentless black bullets as Greg steers the hopeless lifeboat too close to the rocks. A bridge collapse at Hudson Bay, casualties to recover lost in the torrent, swept out to sea... and miles away on the other side of a window, the woman he longs for, trying to forget that he exists.

\*\*\*

THE DOWNPOUR DISTORTING everything as Sam Jackson fixes his eyes on the road and speeds toward the bridge. Slewing too fast around another bend, aching to get home. His heart beating the rhythm of the blades as they wash from side to side, getting faster and faster as he nears the bridge. Slow down, slow down, slow down, they seem to say, but the village-shaped lights pull him onward, twinkling like stars far into the distance through the rippling windscreen.

\*\*\*

DROPS OF PURE midnight falling slant onto neatly mown lawns. They'll be green and lush in the morning but now they're lost lakes of black. Neatly parked cars, lit in patches by all-night porch lights, their colours leaching onto drenched angular drives, and upstairs at number twenty-four, Sonja sleeping. He told her not to wait up, said he'd be home late and not to worry, to take a tablet and go to bed, said he'd see her in the morning for eggs and coffee, and that he loved her.

\*\*\*

THE TUMULT OF rain against black slate roofs, testing every crack for weakness like the dark water it is, feeling with thin fingers into darker places, into black trenches where seawater meets silt, where salty pockets leave pale stains, shrouds of dirty white, where again and again, the tide fetches up its dead.

# The Fleshing of Bones

IT'S DARK WHEN Nick comes home with food and wood. It's our last night at Beach Cottage and though its back to reality tomorrow I'm feeling hopeful. Now that I'm re-writing the nightmares and memories into stories, they seem to be shape-shifting into something I can get past.

The evening is chilly, so Nicko lights the wood burner. I start cooking – a mushroom risotto. When the scent of garlic mixed with woodsmoke and fried mushrooms warms the room, I clear away my writing things from the table so we can eat properly by fire and candlelight. I feel Nick watching me as I work, feel the air thick and warm with his love and appreciation.

'Thanks for making the effort,' he says. 'I feel really good about us going home tomorrow. What Dot said about the writing was bang on, I reckon.

It is making you better.'

He's only skimming the surface though, and I'm not really listening, I'm watching the firelight paint a sunset on his face, thinking about the characters who've been guiding my writing ever since we got here. I can feel them like benign ghosts hovering in the periphery of my imagination, half-formed wraiths waiting to show me something I can almost see. I've had a sense of remembered forgetfulness ever since he got home, like that feeling you get when you walk into a room and forget what it was you went in there for.

We wash the pots and go to bed. I know he's asleep when his breath matches the rhythm of the waves outside. I use the slow ins and outs of his sleep-breathing to empty my mind, then I pick up my pen and notebook, and let them in…

\*\*\*

THE NIGHT IS cold and wet. I dress for the weather – wellington boots and warm overcoat, and start the short walk down to the tideline. As I make my way over the shingle, a strong gust of wind blows a hole in the clouds revealing a pale sliver of new moon. I watch the gannets arrow through the air then slice into the choppy water. I know gannets don't fly after dark, but this is my story and I'm half controlling its construction now.

She appears at the edge where sand meets sea, the beachcomber. She doesn't turn, though she must be able to hear me coming because my boots are crunching over the noisy shingle. I stop beside her, breathing the ozone deep into my lungs as my hair whips backward. She stares ahead, reaches down and presses something into my hand. I don't need to look to know it's a piece of weathered bone that she has collected from the shore.

I curl my fingers around it as I ask, 'But what does it mean?'

'I think you know,' she says, and something starts to stir, not out to sea, but inside my mind, a glimmer immerging like a hazy shadow, like a grey figure rising to the surface, moving toward me. It's Mummy. It's my dead Mummy.

In the real world, I feel my heart beating in my throat, but I don't pay it any attention because I need to stay inside the story. I translate the feelings into words, keeping my mind fixed on the figure as she walks toward the table, sits down, lights four candles. Then the memory shifts, lurching suddenly, and I'm running ahead of her, surefooted in my usual boots, confident at the water's edge despite the rising storm that I love as much as her, that I love because of her. She's seconds behind me, calling my name like it's a game, like we're playing hide-and-seek.

We'd taken a train to the seaside, to Southport I think, had a packed lunch – marmite sandwiches and marzipan fruits – tiny replicas of the real things, oranges, and peaches and apples that looked so real they seemed like magic. We'd built a sandcastle in the wind and rain, had birthday cake – well an iced bun really – in the teashop on the seafront. It had four little candles in it. Just the two of us. She sang my happy birthday and I joined in, giggling as she helped me blow the candles out. It was the last birthday we would ever spend together, and it left no mark, no watery footsteps in the shifting sand, only waves of sorrow crashing back from the hinterland in the margin between worlds where memories are saved or washed away.

Until now.

I am aware that, as I write, my eyes are wet and my mouth is dry, but I block it all out to stay in the story. I run my fictional fingers over the imaginary bone and toss it out, as far into the waves as I can. An arm squeezes my left shoulder and I turn my head to the beachcomber, smiling in something like gratitude because, though my mother's lost and gone forever, I have something vivid and only mine to remember her by. But there's no-one there. I look to the rocks and the mudflats, and back to Beach Cottage, for the familiar figure up close or dotting the horizon, but they're empty of everything, except the gulls and the gannets and the rising wind.

***

I PUT THE pen down for what will be the last time, and go to get myself a drink of water. Tomorrow, when we get home, I'll blow my savings on a laptop and book myself onto a writing course. It'll be the beginning of a new chapter where I'll type, not handwrite my stories – but for now, it's only the handwriting that matters. I go back to bed and read it again and again to anchor the memory. When its secure and I'm sure, I walk to the bedroom window and press my cheek against the cold glass to see outside. It feels strangely solid. I stand and stare for what feels like hours, thinking everything through until a stone-grey dawn lights the horizon. It's not a flat-line horizon this morning, but ruched with irregular pulses, distant peaks and troughs where the tide is turning.

# The Accidental Flash

IT'S THE FIRST day of the creative writing course I signed up for. Distance learning, so I don't have to leave the house. The writing's been great therapy but I'm still a long way away from controlling my bouts of debilitating anxiety. I log into the new tutor group and read the introductions of fifteen strangers, mostly teachers and retired civil servants living all over East Anglia. I add mine. I don't mention mental health or the reasons why I'm doing this. Cyberspace is my ideal environment – you can lie by omission – be the edited highlights of yourself.

No-one else seems to be online in real time, which is a relief, but our tutor has introduced herself already and set us our first creative writing task. Exercise one. Write three six-word stories a la Ernest Hemingway's famous story – *Baby shoes. For sale. Never worn.*

Three years later, writing this, I'll know it probably wasn't written by Hemingway at all, that's just apocryphal. I'll also know that those six words use implication, omission, form (of a classified advertisement), choppy sentences, short and clipped like words are when someone's trying to supress a sob, with full-stops that make pauses like tiny vacuums that readers don't really notice but which they fill up with emotion and their own version of the narrative truth. I'll know all that in the unwritten future, but not yet. Now, reading it just makes me feel sad. I try to channel the sadness instead of drowning in it, processing it for a couple of days as I write many more than six words. When I finally log back on, I check what the others have come up with before summoning the guts to post my own. Everyone else has posted their stories, a few have even given feedback – all positive and upbeat – but my heart is still pounding in my throat when I cut and paste:

> *Dog barks, hackles raised, into nothing;* and
> *Broken heart seeks builder for reconstruction;* and
> *One marriage, two dads, three kids.*

I'm so stressed by having actually put something out there, I go offline for another two days and even then, it takes several swigs of Dutch courage to help me back. But I needn't have worried because everyone, including my tutor thinks they're brilliant, and for the first time – for one fleeting moment – the anxiety morphs into something new. I feel it so strongly it takes my breath away. I haven't heard of flash fiction yet, but I see what the tutor means about small being beautiful and less being more and about imbuing every word and the spaces between with as much intensity as you can. And since intensity is one thing I don't struggle with, I decide that from now on, I'll make every word, every letter, every single moment count, however twitchy I get.

# Historical Elision

ON WEDNESDAY 13<sup>th</sup> August 1969, *Honkey Tonk Woman* was number one.

I'm sitting at my writing desk in front of my new laptop, filling in the fuzzy haze of my early childhood with concrete detail. I sent off for a copy of my mother's death certificate and now I'm Googling her death-day from the safe distance of forty-seven years. Taylor Swift's singing *Blank Space* on Radio 2. This is weird happenstance not a literary device.

My stepmother was such a good woman in very many ways, but when she and Dad first got together, she didn't appreciate anyone mentioning life before their marriage. She didn't make a song and dance about it in front of anybody else, but she'd been my dead mum's best friend and she had a way of making my sister and I feel like *her* loss was greater than ours. The stony looks and sour mouths that our questions elicited made us learn fast enough that our tiny tears were at the bottom of the familial pecking order. We learnt to keep quiet to keep the peace, and little-by-little, our birth mother was elided from family history.

According to the Met Office website, the temperature was 30° when she was having her hysterectomy. By the time she was recovering, a thunderstorm had broken. Did it thunder, I wonder, when the pulmonary embolism struck? Did she see flashes of lightening as she collapsed back into a cloud of white pillows unable to raise the alarm?

Weather-wise her last couple of ordinary days were settled and warm. I imagine the sun falling in dappled patterns through the trees onto the hospital carpark as she locked the door of her blue Ford Anglia. Maybe she listened to *Honky Tonk Woman* on the placky transistor in the kitchen of our little terraced house at 271, Dean Church Lane, before she set off on her final journey.

I expect she knew what was happening at the moment of her death. She was Bolton General

Hospital's youngest ever theatre sister. That's why she was in the privileged position of being lethally alone on an unstaffed side ward. I can see her now in my mind's eye, as the pain took her breath away, her heart breaking as she fought tooth and claw to stay alive for her little daughters. But I'd like to know for sure.

Google's no help. It says there was sectarian violence in Northern Ireland, and that the Apollo 11 astronauts were awarded presidential Medals of Freedom by Richard Nixon.

By the time Bobby Gentry topped the charts in October with *I'll Never Fall in Love Again*, me and our Lesley lived on the other side of town with our paternal grandparents, and Dad and my step-mum were courting. They'd become close consoling each other following their terrible loss. Least that's the story handed down to me. The fuzzy nothing that dulled my early childhood was replaced by a year of sharp clarity and scorch-marked trauma. I still know all the words to all the verses of *I'll Never Fall in Love Again*. I'd sing them to Granny who'd chuckle with delight at the dissonance of hearing a four-year-old singing such world-weary lyrics.

They married on November 6th 1972, when *I Can See Clearly Now* was number one. No need to Google that, I remember every second.

# Getting There

THE DRIVE WAS fine. The A1 was my new best friend, with its skull-toothed juggernauts clattering and snarling round lazy day trippers. Knowing its best to keep busy, the M62 did its bit, with tangled traffic all the stop-start way. The snow was there for me too, swirling over Saddleworth in gripping dust devils.

The hospital megacity gobbled me up. Round-and round I went until I found a place, then a space, then some change, then my registration number which had unremembered itself as I fiddled in front of the high-maintenance machine. On foot, it was easy to find the entrance, so my phylactery fingers and thumbs dialled Dad, like we'd arranged.

We met at Costa and walked to the ward, small-talking to ease the phase-shift into limbo.

The door swung open and he said, 'She's a bit more settled this morning, but late last night she said, "*I think I'm going.*" I say she said it, but she can't really talk, just whispers, so quiet you have to read her lips or put your face that close to hers you're afraid your breath will break her.'

Inside, two pink witches were well bedded in, canting oblivious in broad Boltonian, their Lancashire twang raising no magic.

'Do you wear them incontinence pads Norma? I used to swear by them, but you can't get them ont' NHS, not anymore and they're dead dear.'

'Nowt's cheap now, Ada. You can't get owt for nowt.'

Dad nods them a familiar hello then whispers to me, 'They were at it all night. We don't mind. Your mum gets some peace with her hearing aid turned down.'

Then I spot her, floating tiny over the furthest bed, a hovering mist like dust in a sunbeam – pale particles suspended in the flickering strip light – shifting like morning mist before daytime burns it back to cloud, her version of every shared moment, hanging, drifting. Then she sees me and she's solid, raises a porous hand to lift mine to her lips, smiling a cat's eye smile. It's clear that unsettling smile, so I swallow the salt and bend to kiss her dandelion-clock hair, breathing in.

# The Time-Travellers Step-Daughter

MY STEP-MOTHER'S ALL over the place, hopping from decade to decade. Yesterday, she popped up in 1979 warming tinned potatoes on a camping stove in a layby on the way to Butlins, then five minutes later she was holding hands with me by the sea in Aberystwyth in 1987. Our curly perms held fast, though the wind was brisk. It was just before we went for that meal to Gannett's and got tipsy celebrating my graduation.

Today, she's dancing the Macarena on Instagram with Harry in 2002. Can't remember why.

On Facebook, she's drinking Chablis, sitting at the big oak table at my cottage the night Georgy wouldn't eat his Sunday dinner. She made me cry laughing that night.

'If you won't listen to your mum,' she said,

shooting me a knowing look, 'then listen to your old gran and get that broccoli down your neck. You're way too skinny for my liking. I've seen more meat on a dirty fork.'

It still makes me smile when I look at him looking at her, in that one.

I wonder how long it'll take her to fade?

I'm uploading the last one, now. The one where Dad's helping her out of the wheelchair into the car to go home. Her skin was grey in the autumn sunlight as she turned to say she loved me, her smile gaunt and thin as I clicked for the final time.

I'm going to keep retweeting that one. It's like a sort of short eternity.

# The Waltzers

SOMETIMES I IMAGINE he took us on the waltzers. Just me and our Lesley, at night-time on a rainy Thursday in 1971, when the Michaelmas fair came to Bolton. We'd seen them pitching up when we walked home from school, all noise and clatter on the muddy square of land where the bombed-out back-to-backs used to stand.

If I really let my imagination loose, I can smell the candyfloss and toffee apples; see the coloured lights leaking into the misty drizzle, so the air flashes green and purple and golden. I imagine us clambering inside as the fairground lad yells the instruction to hold on tight. Dad sits in the middle with an arm around both of us and the music starts up. It's so loud we can feel it through the soles of our wellies, and we know all the words to all the songs – *Hot Love* and *Maggie May*. We sing them together, all butterflies and sticky fingers, our eyes blazing in the fairy-lights as we wait for the ride to start.

If he *had* taken us, our waltzer would've trundled slow at first, rattling over the wooden slats, getting faster as it gained momentum, up and down, and round and round, faster and faster until we were whizzing and spinning and screaming in terrified joy, our belly's somersaulting as Dad became our daddy again. We'd have laughed and laughed, clinging onto each other as the centrifugal force pressed us closer together, and that, or some other invisible power would have squished us so close we'd have almost forgotten that one of us was missing – our broken family compressed so tight that for a magical moment we'd have been able to see right inside each other's minds. And even though me and our Lesley were only six and eight, we'd have felt his loss and known how much he still loved our mummy. And he'd have felt our loss too, seen it wasn't a childish nothing that we'd get over in time, but something real and indelible. He'd have understood that we needed to grieve and weep, to let it all out sometimes, instead of keeping it all in, and he'd have seen he shouldn't have cut our mother out so quickly, or let our loss become overwhelmed by my step-mum's because she'd been our dead mother's best friend. He'd have kept photos of her in the house and insisted we stay in contact with our maternal grandparents, given us a grave to visit and flowers to put on top, and answered all our questions so we'd have grown up knowing her middle name and the date she died instead of disappearing her into an angry swirl of hollow nothingness. And in my imagination, when the waltzers stop, we climb out all dizzy and breathless, separate again but somehow still together, and we walk toward a new future holding each other's hands, all the way home.

# Acknowledgements

Thanks to my tutor at the Open University, Katherine Stansfield, for her kindness, expertise and encouragement, and to my ex-OU feedback buddies: Jill Adams, David Artis, Sharon Boyle, Maureen Bowden, June Eglund-Jenkins, Judith Field, Ruth Guthrie, Thomas Malloch, Alli Matthew, Ali McGrane and Simon O'Mahoney.

# About the Author

Jan Kaneen is a mum, wife, sister and daughter who's been a bar maid, betting office cashier, magazine publisher, community development co-ordinator and chief cook and bottle washer for several local charities. She started writing in 2015 at the age of 50, as a sort of mindfulness therapy to help channel her emotions. She now has an MA in Creative Writing from the Open University and her stories have been published widely online and in print, most recently in places like the Bath Flash Anthology, Aesthetica and Comma Press's Dinesh Alirajah Prize Anthology. She's been nominated for Best on the Net, several Pushcarts and Best Microfiction, and one of her flash fictions made the BIFFY 50 2019-20 list. This is her debut Memoir-in-Flash.

# Previous Credits for Flashes in The Naming of Bones

*The Other Side of the Nightmare* was published online in Rhythm and Bone, December 2018.

*We're Going to Pick Daddy Up* was published online in a slightly different form at Retreat West, April 2016.

*Remembering Themselves* was published in print as part of a short story entitled, *The Time-traveller's Daughter*, in the Cheshire Prize for Literature Anthology, 'Patches of Light,' published by Chester University Press, 2016.

*Forget-Me-Not* was published in print in Scribble magazine in 2017 as part of a short story entitled, *Lus y Chooinaght*, which won 3rd prize in their annual short story competition.

Bagsy Blobsy, No Back Answers came second in the 2018 Ely Short Story Competition.

*Waiting* was published online in April 2016 by Molotov Cocktail and in print in The Molotov Cocktail Winners' Anthology II, December 2016.

*Six Things I'll Have Done by the Time You Wake Up* was a finalist in the National Flash Fiction Day drabble competition and was published online by Ellipsis Zine, August 2018.

*Different Ways of Drowning* was published online by Reflex Fiction in June 2018 and in print in the anthology 'The Real Jazz Baby', December 2018.

*Getting There* was published online by Reflex Fiction under the title, *When Holding onto Turns into Letting Go*, August 2018

*The Time-Traveller's Step-Daughter* was published in print in the anthology 'Flash Festival One', Ad Hoc Fiction, 2017.

# More from Retreat West Books

**Winner Most Innovative Publisher 2020**
**Saboteur Awards**

If you've enjoyed this book, we have many more brilliant memoirs, novels and short fiction collections from award-winning authors. Get more information at https://retreatwest.co.uk/books.

## A Song Inside
### *Gill Mann*

'*You are a song inside me now, a melody that stirs and bursts into life when I think of you.*'

In this heart-breaking, thought-provoking and ultimately uplifting memoir, Gill Mann remembers life with her son Sam – a boy and young man who enchanted and infuriated in equal measure. Sam saw colours where others saw grey. He made people feel alive. His unvanquishable spirit sings out as Gill reflects on the joys he brought, the difficulties of his struggles with schizophrenia, and the impact of his death.

Part journal, part journey into the past, and part conversation with Sam, in this beautifully written memoir, Gill thoughtfully and tenderly reveals her relationship with her son, both before and after his death. *A Song Inside* explores universal issues of love and loss to reveal how we can move forward and find happiness again, without leaving behind the people we have lost.

*This beautifully written and tender tribute to a beloved son is full of sadness but also of love. I learned a lot from it.'*

– Cathy Rentzenbrink: writer, journalist and author of the Sunday Times bestselling memoir The Last Act of Love

*'Sam's story is that of lots of young men: different, troubled, beloved and lost. His mother's story, and the family's, is all their own but will raise echoes for many of the process of memory, understanding and resolution.'*

– Libby Purves: radio presenter, journalist and author

## Separated From the Sea

### *Amanda Huggins*

#### *COSTA SHORT STORY AWARD FINALIST –*
#### *COSTA BOOK AWARDS 2018*

*Separated From the Sea* is the debut short story collection from award-winning author, Amanda Huggins.

Crossing oceans from Japan to New York and from England to Havana, these stories are filled with a sense of yearning, of loss, of not quite belonging, of not being sure that things are what you thought they were. They are stories imbued with pathos and irony, humour and hope.

Evie meets a past love but he's not the person she thinks he is; a visit to the most romantic city in the world reveals the truth about an affair; Satseko discovers an attentive neighbour is much more than that; Eleanor's journey on the London Underground doesn't take her where she thought it would.

*This is a writer who knows her craft. Never a word out of place, poignant, sometimes sad, sometimes startling, these stories fit worlds into small spaces. A long awaited debut.*

—Angela Readman – author of
*Don't Try This At Home*

*Amanda's work is well crafted, subtle, and shows a deft hand. I love the way she gets into the psychology of each character, delving into their secret wishes and desires, giving us insights into how and why people act the way they do.*

—A M Howcroft, InkTears – author of
*Nobody Will Ever Love You*

*The reader is transported to many different countries to experience relationships and emotions at the peak of a single moment in the characters' lives. The writing is flawless and carefully shaded, the layers of meaning unfolding elegantly.*

—Joanna Campbell – author of
*When Planets Slip Their Tracks*

*If you want the perfect witness to a crime, Amanda Huggins is your woman. She notices everything about the people, places and the things around her. Colours, temperature, sounds, the lot. And she gets all this down in lovely little stories that spin around in the readers' head, dizzying us with her powerful images of loss, regret and yearning.*

—David Gaffney – author of
*All The Places I've Ever Lived*

## This Is (Not About) David Bowie
### *FJ Morris*

*Every day we dress up in other people's expectations.*

*We button on opinions of who we should be, we instagram impossible ideals, tweet to follow, and comment to judge.*

*But what if we could just let it all go? What if we took off our capes and halos, threw away our uniforms, let go of the future. What if we became who we were always supposed to be?*

*Human.*

*This is (not about) David Bowie. It's about you.*

This Is (Not About) David Bowie is the debut flash fiction collection from F.J. Morris. Surreal, strange and beautiful it shines a light on the modern day from the view of the outsider.

From lost souls, to missing sisters, and dying lovers to superheroes, it shows what it really is to be human in a world that's always expecting you to be something else.

"*In This is (not about) David Bowie, FJ Morris gifts us with a five-part collection of poetry and prose and plays and hybrid works written with daring and verve and a voice that leaps off the page. This book is as inimitable and immersive as Bowie himself, who so wisely said, "The truth is of course is there is no journey. We are arriving and departing all at the same time. "Read this collection, then everything you can find by this exciting author."*

—Kathy Fish, author of
*Wild Life: Collected Works from 2003-2018.*

"*FJ Morris carries off with aplomb the great ask of brilliant flash fiction – that it addresses myriad subjects in a short word count. True, these stories are about David Bowie but also so much more besides. Lovers grow apart, astronauts float in tin cans, men (and women) fall to earth, fledgling explorers take their first tentative steps. Morris poetically shines a spotlight on modern life, boldly embracing different forms where lesser authors can barely manage a beginning, middle and end. A wonderful book, as imaginative as the Jean Genie himself!*"

—Erinna Mettler – author of *Starlings*

## Unprotected
### *Sophie Jonas-Hill*

She's fighting to save everyone else but will she have anything left to save herself? Witty, sharp and sarcastic tattoo artist Lydia's life is imploding. Her long-term relationship has broken down after several miscarriages and she's hiding from her hurt and loss in rage. After a big night out she wakes beside a much younger man who brings complications she could really do without. As her grief about her lost babies and failed relationships spirals out of control, she obsesses about rescuing a wayward teenage girl she watches from her window and gets more involved than she should with her charming but unstable young lover. *Unprotected* is a raw and punchy story of love, family and accepting yourself for who you really are.

*"A raw, viscerally-beautiful gut-punch of a novel about love and loss and heartbreak and hope, and the*

*pain we inflict on each other – and ourselves. Sophie Jonas-Hill is a powerful new voice."*

—Tammy Cohen, author of
*Stop At Nothing*

*"Unprotected is an absorbing, thought-provoking story of betrayal and bravery. Sophie Jonas-Hill probes the darkest corners of modern society with boldness and sensitivity. I loved it!"*

—Ruby Speechley, author of
*Someone Else's Baby*

## Remember Tomorrow
### *Amanda Saint*

Alone. Frightened. Persecuted.

In a not-so-distant future, food is scarce, religion and superstition rule over law, and whispers about witchcraft can be more dangerous than any army. Will herbalist Evie's grandson really carry out his witch-hunting threats?

When society crumbles, activist Evie yearns to build a different kind of life. One of compassion, sustainability and equality. She doesn't expect her own family to oppose her. And when the man responsible for everything wrong in her life suddenly reappears is he there to save her – or to stop her?

*Remember Tomorrow* is a disturbing yet deeply moving portrait of an all-too-possible dystopian future, where family ties can fracture as easily as the world we inhabit – and the damage is not easily repaired.

"A dystopian future that echoes the present times. A reflection of society in a stark, unforgiving mirror. Unsettling, honest and unputdownable."

—Susmita Bhattacharya, author of
*The Normal State of Mind*

"A chilling descent into the chaos that lies in the hearts of men. A searing portrait of a dystopian future where civilisation's thin veneer has been ripped away, and it is women who suffer most as a result. Excellent."

—Paul E. Hardisty, author of *Turbulent Wake*

"I enjoyed every page of Remember Tomorrow. The writing is beautifully emotive and the characters are wonderfully created. It's a world that we hope won't happen, but it's also a world that may not be too far away. Compelling, gripping and at times, deeply unsettling. Remember Tomorrow is a must read and is highly recommended by me."

—Anne Cater, book blogger, and book reviewer for The Daily Express

Printed in Great Britain
by Amazon